# How to Stop Snoring

*Discover How
to Stop Snoring Today*

by Kristof Gustavson

# Table of Contents

Introduction ................................................................... 1

Chapter 1: The Potential Root Cause of Your Snoring .......... 7

Chapter 2: Lifestyle Changes to Eliminate Snoring ............. 13

Chapter 3: Practicing Physical and Breathing Exercises ....... 17

Chapter 4: The Spectrum of Treatment Options ................. 21

Conclusion ..................................................................... 27

# Introduction

If it wasn't for strong love between couples, the number one cause of divorce could have been snoring. Even more gruesome, snoring could be the number one cause of thoughts of murder between couples (don't quote us on this). The annoying thing about snoring is that the snorers themselves aren't aware of the noise they are creating, while the persons around them are definitely fully aware. Sometimes even the neighbors are fully aware. Snoring is a sound that is made involuntarily by someone asleep. Snoring is caused by the vibration of the respiratory tract because the air one breathes in is not flowing properly and naturally. The sound that is produced as a result of the obstruction can range from a mild whimper to something that can rival the roar of a grizzly bear. Snoring is an often mocked and laughed at condition, but it can also be very dangerous.

The problem with snoring is not so much the noise but that it could be indicating a bigger underlying condition that could be affecting the individual. One of these conditions is sleep apnea, which is characterized by short, shallow and infrequent breathing during sleep. A person suffering with sleep apnea will stop breathing at irregular intervals, and these times could last up to a half a minute. This condition is downright scary to the sufferer's sleep partner, and often the person will have to keep on checking that he or she is still alive. Yes, sleep apnea can be fatal, and if a person snores, it could indicate that the person is suffering from this problem.

Most people have snored at least once in their lifetime, but there are a few that snore on a regular basis. Statistics show that at least 30% of American adults snore and, in some countries and other demographics, the percentage of snorers can be as high as 50%. In television shows and movies, men are the ones more often portrayed snoring and women less so. This mirrors real life, as it is shown that about 24% of men snore compared to 13.8% of women. This number increases as people age, with 60% of men over the age of 60 being snorers, while only 40% of women of the age of 60 do. Luckily for most people, there are remedies and treatments for snoring. If you or your partner snores, it is recommended that you visit a doctor to discover if there are underlying causes of the problem.

In this book, we'll discuss snoring some more and see what really causes snoring. Then we'll discuss how those who suffer from this condition can find relief for themselves and those around them.

© Copyright 2015 by Miafn LLC - All rights reserved.

This document is geared towards providing reliable information in regards to the topic and issue covered. The publication is sold with the idea that the publisher is not required to render accounting, officially permitted, or otherwise, qualified services. If advice is necessary, legal or professional, a practiced individual in the profession should be ordered.

- From a Declaration of Principles which was accepted and approved equally by a Committee of the American Bar Association and a Committee of Publishers and Associations.

In no way is it legal to reproduce, duplicate, or transmit any part of this document in either electronic means or in printed format. Recording of this publication is strictly prohibited and any storage of this document is not allowed unless with written permission from the publisher. All rights reserved.

The information provided herein is stated to be truthful and consistent, in that any liability, in terms of inattention or otherwise, by any usage or abuse of any policies, processes, or directions contained within is solely and completely the responsibility of the recipient reader. Under no circumstances will any legal responsibility or blame be held against the publisher for any reparation, damages, or monetary loss due to the information herein, either directly or indirectly.

Respective authors own all copyrights not held by the publisher.

The information herein is offered for informational purposes solely, and is universal as so. The presentation of the information is without contract or any type of guarantee assurance.

The trademarks that are used are without any consent, and the publication of the trademark is without permission or backing by the trademark owner. All trademarks and brands within this book are for clarifying purposes only and are the owned by the owners themselves, not affiliated with this document.

# Chapter 1: The Potential Root Cause of Your Snoring

Snorers breathe through their mouths when they are asleep, which deviates from the natural way of breathing – through our nose. When we breathe normally through the nose, the air passes over the palate into the throat without any obstruction. But when we breathe through the mouth, the air doesn't pass through the necessary breathing mechanisms that ensure the air enters the pharynx and lungs smoothly and cleanly. This creates large vibrations in the soft tissue. When we sleep, the muscles in the pharynx and larynx are supposed to be relaxed, but in snorers, they are not as relaxed causing tension and obstruction. Snoring is caused by many different conditions, which include obesity, snoring, and old age.

Snoring is often a condition on its own, but it could also be a symptom of another more serious condition. One of these conditions is called sleep apnea. Sleep apnea is a sleep disorder where the respiratory tract gets completely blocked during irregular intervals, causing the cessation of breathing. These pauses could last from 5 seconds, to as long as a few minutes. They can occur several times up to 30 times in an hour. This is very dangerous to the individual, and can be very scary for the individual's partner, as sleep apnea can be fatal. When the person starts breathing again after a pause in breathing, they often make a loud noise which can either wake them up or wake their partners up. Because the person keeps waking up, they will find that they are tired in the mornings or find it very difficult to wake up in the mornings.

Persons who suffer from sleep apnea find that they are lethargic during the daytime, and will often be miserable as they go about the day. If you find you are tired throughout the day, you should visit a sleep doctor to get yourself diagnosed. A 1993 study shows that at least one in every 15 Americans suffered from at least moderate sleep apnea.

If you go to a sleep doctor, they will perform what is known as a formal sleep study, or a *polysomnography*. The doctor will find if cessation of breath does occur, and they will then see how many of these events happen per hour of sleep. If apnea events occur for less than 15 times in an hour, then it is known as mild obstructive sleep apnea. If it occurs between 15 and 30 times per hour, it is known as moderate obstructive sleep apnea. If it occurs for more than 30 times per hour, then it is known as sever obstructive sleep apnea.

If you feel tired throughout the day but don't want to do to the doctor unless you are really sure, what you could do is make an audio recording of yourself while you sleep. It is best to use a digital recorder or your phone, so that you can quickly manipulate it on a computer. Once you have a recording, use an audio software such as Audacity to look at sound waves of the recording. Look for any special events, as these places will have higher peaks than others. Do this a minimum of three nights, and compare results. If you find yourself taking deep and sharp breaths more than 5 times per hour during sleep, then it might be time to visit a sleep doctor.

Unfortunately and even more frighteningly, obstructive apnea is not the only kind of apnea you want to look out for. There is also central apnea, which is a neurological problem. While the chance of death from obstructive apnea is not very high, central apnea can cause psychological damage and even sudden death. When central apneas occur, the parts of our brain that regulate breathing during sleep stop working all of a sudden, and the parts of the brain that are supposed to detect increased levels of carbon dioxide due to the individual not breathing properly do not work. Normal breathing would resume on its own, but there are times when the lack of oxygen is too much for the body to recover from. Do not panic, as the chances of a person acquiring this condition is rare, and the chance of someone dying from this condition is rarer. Consult a doctor for an examination and proper diagnosis.

Another cause of snoring is a person's weight. A person is more likely to snore the more they are overweight. Excess body weight is more of a problem in men than in women where snoring is concerned. Why is that? Well it all comes down to how differently men and women store fatty tissues. Men usually store fat in their abdomens and necks, while women store fat in their pelvic regions and thighs. Because there is more fat in the throat regions of overweight people, they will find that it is harder to breathe because the fat is allowing less room to breathe. It is believed that a man that has a collar size over 16.5 will have a higher chance of snoring.

Another cause of snoring is smoking and alcohol. It is found that smokers are twice more likely to snore than non-smokers. This is because the smoke and tar from the cigarette irritates the nasal mucosa. Smoking can affect non-smokers as well by second-hand smoke.

Another cause of snoring is age. Of course, age itself is not the problem, but it is the conditions and changes that come with age that causes snoring in the first place. This is one of the few causes of snoring that we can't reverse, well that's until we find the fountain of youth, literally or figuratively. Until then, there are some safeguards which can be implemented to try and prevent snoring.

Finally, snoring can be caused by allergic reactions or illnesses like the flu. Because your nose is blocked during the night, and your throat is producing more mucus than normal during these times, you may find that breathing is obstructed. The obstruction then causes a vibration to occur in the throat, which causes the snoring sounds that we all loathe.

Now that we understand the different causes of snoring, we can move to better understand how we can reduce it and better yet, get rid of it. Some of these ways involves the taking of drugs, or using special devices that encourage more positive air flow. But in most cases, snoring can be reduced and cured by changing one's lifestyle.

# Chapter 2: Lifestyle Changes to Eliminate Snoring

Getting rid of your snoring or reducing it comes down to changing a lot of habits, small and large. First of these habits that you may have to change is your sleeping habits. When you snore, the soft palate at the back of your throat and your upper throat close in on each other, restricting the passage of air. Because the air is restricted, the air is sort of forced, which causes a vibration in your throat, and the resulting snoring. You can however reverse this effect by sleeping on your sides or on your belly instead of sleeping on your back, which makes it much harder for the soft palate to collapse on your upper throat. If you prefer to sleep on your back, then it is also helpful to use multiple pillows to prop yourself up. When your head is elevated, your tongue is less likely to block your respiratory pathway. You should also consider elevating the head of your bed, but only if you sleep alone or if your sleep partner agrees.

Another way to ensure that your snoring is reduced is by having a regular sleep pattern. Many of us have irregular sleep schedules, which causes many problems apart from just snoring. You can treat your snoring by getting a regular sleep schedule, including having a regular bed time. When a person doesn't sleep properly, they find that they often crash, and when crashes occur, they fall into a very deep and intense sleep. This deep and intense sleep then causes the muscles in the throat to be more relaxed than usual, which could cause snoring. It is advised that one must have at least six hours of sleep, but the recommended is 7-8 hours. It may be hard for those who have very busy work lives, but you should try to get in as much sleep as you can at night time. Napping is also good to make up for any sleep hours you missed during the night time.

Make sure that you reduce your alcohol and caffeine intake as well. Not only can these two mess up your sleep patterns, but people who consume these substances regularly have a higher chance of snoring. Avoid other things that may be making your situation worse, such as sleeping pills and fatty foods. As was said earlier, fats can press down on the respiratory tract, which can cause snoring. Also, don't have large meals, especially before bed. If you find that you are overweight, then you may have to try and lose weight which we will talk about later.

A lot of snoring is caused by allergies, hence it is important that you keep yourself away from all allergens and keep your area clean. If you breathe in too many allergens such as dust, pollen, mildew, and dander, your throat will react negatively. Spend time to eliminate these threats by vacuuming your area, especially if your bedroom has a carpet. Wash your sheets and clothes regularly as well, as you will want them to be clean as possible. If you have pets, then you may want to quit sleeping with them or stop letting them sleep in your room.

Finally, in all of this ensure that you talk to the right people, especially your partner and your doctor. Your doctor will guide you with steps which you can take to help you end snoring. You should also talk to your partner and hear what they have to say about your condition. Let them know that they have a role in reducing this condition as well.

# Chapter 3: Practicing Physical and Breathing Exercises

As mentioned, obesity is one of the major causes of snoring. But did you know that you can do breathing and other types of exercises to correct your snoring problem as well? Tongue stretching is one of the most recommended exercises. It is important to do this type of exercise as your tongue is involved in obstructing the respiratory pathway while you sleep. Those with a more relaxed tongue during sleep often have a louder snore. By conditioning your tongue with the use of stretches, you can minimize the chance that your tongue will become too relaxed when you sleep. Stretching your tongue also gives your throat a good workout as well. You stretch your tongue by upward and downward movements, trying to get to your nose and chin as much as possible.

Another exercise that you can do is the alternate nostril breath exercise. This is important as one of the reasons why snorers breathe through their mouths is due to the fact that their nasal passages are blocked. However, if you condition your body in the right way of breathing, you can increase the probability of breathing through your nose even though blockage may occur. When you practice alternate nostril breathing, you will breathe deeply, which trains your body to breathe deeper at nights. You can do this exercise by closing one nostril, and then inhaling deeply through the other. Hold your breath, then slightly close your other nostril and exhale.

Do this the other way around and keep alternating. It is good to do this about 10 times per day.

Protruding your lower jaw is another exercise that you could do. When you sleep, your lower jaw and tongue are the primary culprits involved in obstructing the airways. By training your jaw to stay out, you can reduce this problem. You will have to do this on a regular basis, for about 10 seconds each. It is recommended that you do this 10 to 15 times a day.

Finally, it is important that you lose weight. Not only can you lose weight through your diet, but you can lose weight through exercise. You may be tired with seeing this advice repeated, and it may just be a cliché, but exercise is very important. It seems to be the cure for just about everything, but it truthfully may be, as exercise involves the movement and conditioning of different muscles. Even working out muscles that are not directly connected to your throat muscles such as your arms and legs, will indirectly tone your throat muscles as well.

# Chapter 4: The Spectrum of Treatment Options

There are many types of medication and treatment procedures and devices that can be used to treat snoring. In most cases, the first step in treating snoring is through the changing of habits and behaviors. Some of these were already discussed previously, such as changing the way that we sleep, reducing the chances of exposure to allergens, exercising more, and quitting smoking and drinking.

A doctor may recommend the use of a continuous positive airway pressure device (CPAP) or the use of an automatic airway pressure device (APAP). These devices ensure that the respiratory pathway remains open. There is a CPAP machine which generates the best air pressure which is required to keep the airways open during sleep. The difference between CPAP and APAP is that the APAP machine will automatically determine the best air pressure for the person to breathe properly while the CPAP will have to be manually configured. These machines are not cheap, and the use of them could run a bill of up to $1000 dollars a year. Also, as you can imagine, these devices are not very comfortable to use. The patient may even experience side effects with the use of this machine such as skin and nose irritations resulting in a dry nose and mouth, sore gums or nosebleeds. Because of this, don't expect to use this in the long-term, as most people only use it on a short-term basis.

The louder noises during snoring are usually caused by the tongue falling back into the throat. This can be treated with the use of neurostimulation. This procedure uses a device which sends a mild electrical pulse at the back of the tongue so that the tongue won't block your airway. It is a kind of maintenance treatment, the patient will have to do it every time they are about to sleep. Don't worry though, it doesn't hurt at all. The use of tongue guards can also reduce the chance of your tongue blocking the air passage. The jaw and tongue is often too far back when sleeping, and a guard will temporarily or permanently advance the lower jaw. This is only for certain snorers though, and it is important to see a doctor before considering the use of any treatment. There are other mandibular splints which pull the tongue and jaw forward.

The Pillar Procedure, which is fairly new, involves the use of three or so dacron strips and inserting them into the soft palate. Dacron strips are used in permanent sutures. The soft palate gets more rigid as a result of these insertions, which reduces the chance of snoring and sleep apnea. This procedure can either be used alone or combined with other procedures.

There are drugs that can help reduce the intensity of snoring. These drugs include pseudoephedrine and domperidone, which are rising in popularity as effective treatments. There are also drugs that were developed for sleep apnea that may be used by snorers, such as zolpidem and triazolam. If you have sinus problems and allergies, you could reduce the snoring problem yourself by taking a decongestant or an antihistamine. These drugs will clear your nasal passages so that you breathe through your nose instead of your mouth.

The last option that doctors might advise you to consider is surgery. Some of these procedures are used in sleep apnea patients as well. One of the more popular throat surgeries is uvulopalatopharyngoplasty, or UPP. This involves the removal of tissues in the back of the throat, which includes the pharynx and the uvula. These are last resort options, as there is a chance that this type of procedure will cause adverse side effects. One of these is a more dangerous condition, which is caused by the scarring of tissues resulting from the surgery. When these tissues scar, they swell and diminish the airspace of the pharynx, sometimes even worse than before. This is very rare, and it is very hard to tell what makes internal tissues react to scarring in this way. Luckily, the chance of this turning into something fatal is slim.

Another surgical procedure is called radiofrequency ablation, which applies radiofrequency and heat to the soft tissue at the back of the throat which causes scarring. Unlike the UPP, the scarring does not result in swelling, but instead results in a hardening of the area. This procedure is done in several treatment sessions, and last about an hour each. This method is effective in reducing the effect of snoring, but it does not eliminate it.

Surgery is 95% effective at curing snoring, and the most effective procedure of them all is the maxillomandibular advancement procedure. Here, the lower jaw is brought forward, which decreases the chance of the tongue blocking the airspace. This procedure is also used to treat sleep apnea. Studies are still continuing on the effectiveness and the side effects of surgery. Many believe that surgery could cause death in that the anesthetics that are used remain in the system for days afterward, and if the person has central apnea problem, then it can increase the risk of suddenly dying in their sleep. Also, surgical procedures on this part of the body result in higher risk of swelling. However, these swellings resolve eventually and a doctor will typically prescribe drugs that can reduce these effects.

# Conclusion

The vast majority of the world's population has snored at least once in their lifetime, since the obstruction of the air passage during sleep is not uncommon. However, there are those who suffer from this condition often and it affects the quality of sleep for themselves and those around them. Some people who snore wake up the next morning fatigued, miserable and irritable, mostly because they aren't breathing right throughout the night and their sleep is disturbed often. This is heightened when a person suffers from sleep apnea. However, the person who usually suffers the most is the one who has to sleep beside the snorer through the night.

If you are past middle age, if you are male, if you have had nasal and sinus problems in the past, if you are overweight, if you smoke or drink, or if you lie on your back, you are more likely to snore. Apart from age and sex, you can just about fix many of the common causes of snoring. Once you take steps to correct your problem, you will find that you sleep much better, and both you and your partner will be much happier.

Finally, I'd like to thank you for purchasing this book! If you found it helpful, I'd greatly appreciate it if you'd take a moment to leave a review on Amazon. Thank you!

Printed in Great Britain
by Amazon